Publisher's Note: This is a work of fiction. Names, characters, places, and incidents are a product of the author's imagination. Locales and public names are sometimes used for atmospheric purposes. Any resemblance to actual people, living or dead, or to businesses, companies, events, institutions, or locales is completely coincidental.

This book is not intended as a substitute for the medical advice of physicians. The reader should regularly consult a physician in matters relating to his/her health and particularly with respect to any symptoms that may require diagnosis or medical attention. (*health, alternative healing*) Before beginning any new exercise program it is recommended that you seek medical advice from your personal physician.

#TheSprintDiet

http://workoutkingrule.blogspot.com/

My Story

If you're looking for someone that's going to use fancy words and bullshit to sell you on a good comprehensive workout than you've come to the wrong place. If you're looking for someone who's going to use periods and commas in the right place than you've come to the wrong place. This is going to be straightforward and to the point. I'm not going to sit here and bullshit you. I'm not going to give you information that didn't work for me because that would be stupid and completely misleading.

Let me tell you my story. I was a regular attractive young guy and then I got in a relationship. Once that happened I gain an extremely large amount of weight. The next thing you know I'm not in a relationship anymore and I'm 50 pounds heavier. I've never had to lose weight a day in my life. I've never had to watch my calories. I've never had to exercise. All this shit was completely new to me. If I had a time machine I would go back and say hey dumbass just sprint.

Sprinting makes perfect sense it's the most effective workout in the world and it only takes you a couple of minutes. Sprinting just makes common sense. I tried every single one of those machines in the gym. I tried the elliptical the bike and of course the fucking treadmill. Now for anybody who's been in the gym for longer than ah month you've seen people use these machines. Ask yourself do they look any different? Has anything changed about them whatsoever? Most likely not! That's not to say those machines don't work but if your goal is to lose weight than those machines are not the answer. They say if you want to lose weight the best way to do it is to diet. If you workout for about a month you may have lost about 10 pounds on the treadmill but gained 10 pounds of muscle so when you get on the scale you're going to weigh the same. Most people don't understand that your body is composed of muscle and fat so they're going to think they didn't lose any weight. Most likely they're going to give up because they think working out isn't effective. I've given up many of times and I have the stretch marks to prove it but once I discovered sprinting I started to understand how the body works. You might be an individual who is composed of 50% body fat and 50% muscle. That's not good! That means you're extremely overweight. For men anything above 30% is high body fat. 21-30% is excess fat. 13-20% is moderately lean. 9-12% body fat is lean. 5-8% body fat is ultra lean but anything below 5% is risky because you have to have some fat to protect internal organs, provide energy, and regulate hormones. For women it's different. Anything above 40% is risky high body fat. 31-40% is excess fat. 23-30% is moderately lean. 19-22% body fat is lean. 15-18% is ultra lean and anything below 15% is risky low body fat.

If you want to change your body fat you have to increase the amount of muscle you have in your body. When you increase the amount of muscle you have in your body you burn fat more efficiently therefore making your day even more effective. You want to increase the amount of calories you burn at rest. That means you want to increase the amount of calories you burn doing absolutely nothing but sitting on your ass. This is called the resting metabolic rate. Your resting metabolic rate is highly affected by your muscle and your mitochondria. So what increases the amount of muscle that you have and increases the amount of mitochondria you have? If your answer is sprinting you're correct! As a matter of fact sprinting is the only exercise that can burn fat and build muscle at the same time. I realized that the three hours I was spending on the elliptical was a complete and utter waste of time I could literally get the same results by sprinting for 3 minutes.

The Benefits Of Sprinting

Sprinting will help you build strength and power in your fast-twitch fibers. Fast twitch fibers are what you use when you punch as fast and as hard as you can. You use your fast twitch fibers when you exert yourself as hard as you possibly can in any exercise. It's basically the number one muscle that you would use in a flight or fight situation. Sprinting also increases protein synthesis pathways by as much as 230% helping you build stronger muscles faster. Protein synthesis is probably one of the most important factors to building muscle.

When you're on a treadmill or ah elliptical you have absolutely no idea what it is that your body is burning. You could be burning muscle.

You could be burning sugar. You could be burning carbohydrates. When you're sprinting you're definitely burning fat sprinting isn't going to change the number on the scale but it is going to change the number on your measuring tape. You lose body fat not body mass that's because your body more effectively burns fat when it's exerting its self at a higher intensity. To put it is numbers your body burns fat better when you're giving your workout 47 to 64% effort. Basically the more intense the workout is the more likely it is that you're burning fat. Less intensity increases the likelihood of you burning various other fuel sources in your body. So if you're a person with a lot of fat on your body that's the most dominant fuel source available so when you're exerting yourself at a high intensity of course your body is going to reach for it's most dominant fuel source.

Sprinting literally trains the body to burn fat for fuel so you can preserve muscle glycogen and prolong your workout. This is why it increases your endurance so significantly. If you are a long distance runner you want to sprint to increase your energy and endurance. By going at max speed you amplify your oxygen uptake and when you do that you increase the time it takes for fatigue to set in. To put it simple you increase the amount of mitochondria in your body and mitochondria is responsible for energy production. Mitochondria takes fat, sugar, muscle, carbohydrates, and other resources in your body and converts them into ATP. ATP is the energy currency of your body so the more mitochondria you have the more efficient your body is at creating energy. The more efficient your body is at creating energy the longer you can run, the longer you can jump, and the longer you can lift.

Sprinting also increases the speed and power of an individual because it's essentially speed training. Sprinting is exactly what a track star does to train. Track stars sprint to increase the strength of their fast twitch muscles, which are responsible for their speed. So the more you sprint the faster you become. Sprinting also lowers blood pressure because it increases the power of your fast-twitch muscles, which improve heart function significantly. Exerting that explosive energy will make your heart pump harder which will strengthen it and decrease the likelihood of you contracting a heart disease. Sprinting saves time because you only need to do 2 minutes and 30 seconds of it a day to receive the same results that you would get from about an hour to 30 minutes of aerobic exercise. It also builds mental toughness as well because they're going to be times that you want to give up. Overcoming this feeling will strengthen your resolve.

Sprinting is probably the hardest form of exercise that you possibly can do because it's the most demanding form of exercise there is. Still since you don't have to do very much of it sprinting has the benefit of saving you a significant amount of time. You don't have to worry about working it around your work schedule. It won't get in the way of you taking care of your children. You don't need to call a baby sitter. It literally is something you can do right before you go to bed or right when you wake up in the morning.

For 2 minutes and 30 seconds of exercise a day you can reduce your stress. When you sprint you produce a significant amount of endorphins, which are like your body's natural painkillers. You'll get a strong euphoric sensation from this type of exercise.

The best way to describe it is to call it what it is, it's a high probably one of the best highs you can get without using a substance. Sprinting improves glucose control, which helps you regulate your insulin so that you don't get high cholesterol, high blood pressure, or high blood sugar, and of course abdominal body fat. It does this because it completely drains the body of glycogen, which than releases the sugar stored inside of our muscles.

Now for the Holy Grail of sprinting, it is the most effective exercise on abdominal belly fat! Number one it makes your abdominals contract more than any other exercise. Number two it improves glucose control, which is a major cause of abdominal body fat. To put it simple sprinting helps you burn fat and prevent new fat from forming. Sprinting increases your energy level and your endurance. By increasing energy and endurance you can work out longer and harder. By increasing mitochondria you also increase your metabolic rate, which means you burn more fat at rest. It's literally the most effective exercise you could possibly do and it doesn't take you any time to do at all.

So why is no one sprinting? Most people don't even know about it, it's not the most famous form of exercise. Unlike the elliptical, stair climber, treadmill, and bike sprinting doesn't really have a big voice. Athletes are the exception because they understand the benefits of sprinting. This is why they're in better physical shape than everyone else on the planet. Sprinting is why Usain Bolt is the fastest man in the world. It's why all your favorite basketball players are able to play non-stop without passing out. It's why long distance runners continue to set records. It's the one exercise that takes you from being fit to being an athlete to being an Olympian.

Beginners Guide

Now this is where plenty of mistakes are made. When you first start sprinting you don't want to over exert yourself. The best method is to do six ten second sprints that one minute. Make sure you go full out I mean no holds bars. If you sit down after the sprint and you still have energy left than you didn't sprint. Sprinting should leave you absolutely exhausted. There shouldn't be anything left in the tank. If there is than you need to sprint harder. You might need to increase the amount of time that you sprint. If you still have energy after ten seconds I would suggest four fifteen-second sprints. By sprinting for a minute every single day you'll start to notice the changes in your body. Your energy will start increasing and your stress will go down.

Before I go on any longer I probably should explain the stress that sprinting can have on your joints. This is why you should never sprint on cement. Even Olympic sprinters don't run on cement. To be honest they don't train on the track every single day because the track is an incredibly hard surface. Most sprinters run on grass or dirt. The smartest thing you could do is run on sand it's a very difficult surface to move on and the added drag makes the sprint that much more effective not to mention the surface isn't aggressive on your joints at all. Me personally I sprint on carpet usually I'll get a yoga mat and place it on top of my carpet than I'll sprint in place. Sprinting in place is very effective to be honest it's just as effective as a moving sprint. As long as you exert yourself to complete exhaustion you're on the right track.

Let me explain my process in better detail. You can either do it my way or you can find your own way of doing it. Just make sure the surface you're sprinting on is soft. First I lay my yoga mat down on the floor and fold it in half. Second I turn my fan on and face it towards my resting place so basically the spot I'm going to sit after I do my sprint. I place my water bottle right next to my rest area because you have to remain hydrated especially when you're exerting this amount of energy. If you don't stay hydrated it could be dangerous. I take my computer out and go to Google. I type in timer. Google has a timer app that appears in the search engine. You can either set ah alarm or you can use the stopwatch feature.

For this exercise I use the stopwatch feature. When I'm ready I press start and than I immediately start pumping my arms and legs as fast as I possibly can. I don't lift my knees up super high because that lowers your speed a lot. I want to move my legs as fast as I can so keeping my knees below my waist is important. I make sure to keep up right so that my core is stabilized. By keeping upright I make sure that I get the maximum abdominal benefit from the exercise. If you lean forward too much your core isn't holding up your upper body, which means it's not being properly worked out. Make sure you run on the balls of your feet not your heels. Now staying in the same spot isn't something I'm very good at. I usually end up all over the room. You want to stabilize your position so that you stay in the same spot especially because you don't want to move off the yoga mat. At no point do you want to decrease your speed you have to be at full intensity for the entire 10-second duration of the sprint otherwise it's not a sprint. Once I see the stopwatch reach 10 seconds I immediately sit down. Never count out the seconds you'll get it wrong ever time use some sort of stopwatch.

The breeze of the fan helps me to relax and recover as I drink some water. Since you're new to this exercise you want to rest until you're ready for the next run. You don't want to put a time limit on your rest. Once you become more acquainted with ten second sprints you want to keep your rest periods down to about 30 seconds unless your doing 30 second sprints than your going to need two minutes of rest. In the beginning you might rest from 1 minute to 2 minutes or even 5 minutes in between each sprint. Now when I'm done with my 6th sprint I'm usually completely wiped out I try to recover by drinking plenty of water and resting until I'm ready to move again. The feeling that I have after my 6th sprint is a combination of fatigue and euphoria. It's a weird kind of high that I can't really explain but the more you sprint the better the high gets. Now you want to do these one-minute sprints everyday for at least 1 week than you want to try to add more sprints to your regiment. The beginning goal is to go from 6 to 12 ten second sprints so you're doing a total of 2 minutes of sprints everyday. Your secondary goal is to go from 12 ten-second sprints to eight 15 second sprints, which is still two minutes but you've increased how long you can run per sprint which is incredibly important. You can stretch before and after you do this sprinting routine. I personally don't that's probably because I sprint in place I don't sprint on a track or outdoors so there isn't too much impact on my joints. For me sprinting in place is much more demanding than an actual moving sprint probably because I can move my body faster when I'm sprinting in place compared to a moving sprint.

You want to make sure you move your arms back and forth from about your ear to your hip. The faster you pump your arms the faster your body will move. When I first started sprinting after about the third day pretty much all the muscles in my body became sore I had to take about two to three days off and than start sprinting again but after that I never became sore again. That happened because the various muscles that I was using to conduct the sprint hadn't been used through all of my other workouts especially not at that intensity. I had extreme muscle soreness in my back which was surprising to me at first until I took into account the intensity in which I was swinging my arms they were going all the way back than all the way forward so I was activating muscles in my back that I had never activated before. If this beginner s*** is to easy for you start off at an intermediate lever. If that's easy for you start off at ah advance level.

Intermediate Guide

Once you can do eight 15-second sprints than you've reached the intermediate level. Now when most people reach this level they always want to start using different devices when they sprint. People want to get on the treadmill and sprint, which by the way is horrible for your joints especially for your knees. Do not sprint on the treadmill! Sprinting on the treadmill is incredibly dangerous! You never want to sprint on a hard moving surface nothing about that sounds like a good idea. Make sure you stay away from surfaces that can be strenuous on your joints. Some individuals want to sprint on bikes this I would recommend because there's virtually no impact whatsoever. The only difference from sprinting on a bike and sprinting in place is that there's no arm movement so you might be able to sprint on a bike longer than you would be able to sprint in place. Some individuals want to sprint using the elliptical. Elliptical sprinting is not intermediate sprinting you're not ready to sprint on an elliptical yet.

If you are on an intermediate level you have just a few goals. The first goal is to go from eight 15-second sprints to six 20-second sprints. So you'll still be doing two-minute sprints you'll just be increasing the duration of each individual sprint. Once you get to this point you want to hold it here for about a week. After a week you want to add another sprint to the equation so you're doing 7 twenty-second sprints. The next week you want to do eight. The week after that you want to do 9. Once you reach nine 20 second sprints you've reached the advanced level. Now don't worry if you're not capable of following this week by week plan go at your own pace. As long as you wind up doing 9 twenty second sprints you'll be okay. Take your time and give your body rest. Once you're doing nine 20 second sprints you're doing 3 minutes of sprinting every single day that's advanced level s*** right there. Give yourself a huge pat on the back for having that much power because that's what sprint accomplishments are advancement in power. Your body is literally becoming more powerful every single day because you're increasing the amount of mitochondria in your body, which means your energy levels are going up every single day.

Advance Sprinting

Now there are many goals once you get to advanced sprinting. First and foremost you want to go from nine 20-second sprints to six 30-second sprints. You'll still be doing 3 minutes of sprinting but you'll be increasing your time per sprint. Now this might be the last time you increase your time per sprint. 30 seconds to me should be the max. Some people can do 60 seconds sprints if you can reach that point than by all means go there. 60-second sprints would be a 400-meter dash. 30-second sprints would be 250-meter dash. 20-second sprints would be a 200-meter dash. 10-second sprints would be a 100-meter dash. If 30 seconds becomes easy than increase your time to 35, 40, 45, 50, 55, and than 60. Just three sixty-second sprints is murder but you could max out at 6 sixty-second sprints. Mind you that is insanity six 30-second all out sprints is plenty especially if you're sprinting in place because you don't have to lift your knees up incredibly high. Lifting your knees up incredibly high reduces your speed so of course you're sprint will last longer. Now the last thing you want to do is add one more 30-second sprint to your regiment maxing you out at 3 minutes and 30 seconds. That's seven 30-second sprints. Once you reach this point you're truly ready for some advanced level sprinting.

You're probably reading this and thinking that this sounds crazy because 3 minutes and 30 seconds of exercise doesn't sound like a long time but once you actually start sprinting you'll look at this section differently. To be honest once you start sprinting this might even seem impossible. Having this level of energy will make you feel like you're 15 again, which makes sense because mitochondria is directly related to aging.

Mitochondria are an entirely separate organism they has their own DNA our relationship with them begin a long, long, long, time ago. Do to free radicals the communication between our two genomes brakes down over time causing major problems. The best way to prevent this from happening is to sprint. Sprinting is the most effective way to increase the body's mitochondrial function keeping you energetic young and healthy.

Now that you've reached a truly advanced level with sprinting you can start to add some extra spice to your workout the first thing I would recommend trying is leg weights. Leg weights are incredibly effective at increasing the difficulty of your sprint workout. I would recommend that you do not go over 5 pounds on each leg. Once you go over 5 pounds on each leg you risk injury because the heavier the leg weights are the more they move around. I usually put 2.5 pounds on each leg it's a lot easier to manage and I don't have to worry about the leg weights moving around. Even five pounds on each leg can be tricky if you don't have the right kind of leg weights. The increased resistance really makes the workout much more rewarding. Most people are not able to adjust to having leg weights on because it creates an imbalance between the arms and the legs if this is the case than you want to wear arm weights as well. Make sure that they are the exact weight otherwise you'll throw off your equilibrium. So 2.5 pounds on each leg and 2.5 pounds on each arm adding a total of 10 pounds to your body.

Now if you're doing moving sprints than a weight vest would be effective but if you were sprinting in place a weighted vest wouldn't be very effective. Sprinting on sand is incredibly effective it's probably one of the most difficult sprint workouts you can do and adding leg weights, arm weights, and ah weighted vests would make it even more difficult. That's real advanced sprint training. Hill sprints are a favorite amongst athletes just make sure the hill you're running up isn't concrete. Run up a grass hill or a dirt hill.

Now all these things are fine and all but the most advanced form of sprint training in my opinion is elliptical sprint training. Not only is it the most advanced form of sprint training but it's also the safest form of sprint training because it's virtually zero impact. Elliptical sprinting is resistance sprinting. You can continue to increase the resistance on the machine making it more and more difficult for you to sprint making the workout that much more effective. You want to turn the resistance up until it's actually difficult for you to move than you sprint your ass off. You want it to be so difficult that you can only sprint for 10 seconds. You want to do 6 ten second sprints. You want to continue doing this until this resistance level becomes easy for you. Than you want to increase your time following the beginner, intermediate, and advance formula all over again. This kind of workout was literally a life-changer for me. I went from 250 pounds 50% body fat to 200 pounds 13% body fat and all I did was work out for 3 minutes and 30 seconds a day.

It's very important to know what your body is made of. You want to measure your resting metabolic rate and you're fat and muscle content. The best way to do that is to use the bod pod. Look up the bod pod online and find out if one is near you. Your gym might already have one it might cost you anywhere from $40 to $60 to use it but it's incredibly worth it. It's like getting a detailed diagnostic on your bodies composition. Actually it is getting a detailed diagnostic of your body's composition.

The Kettlebell Cleanse

Sprinting is incredibly powerful still if you combine it with weight training it becomes that much more powerful. Now most people don't have time to go to the gym to use complex weight training equipment that's why the best solution is to use the Kettlebell. The Kettlebell is a tested and proven tool not to mention it's one of the only forms of weight training that burns and extremely large amount of calories. 3 hours of kettlebell training would burn 3600 calories that's a pound + 100 calories. The kettlebell works out every single inch of the body so you don't have to worry about getting any other machine. It can do everything that all the complex machines in the gym can do and it's only one tool. You just have to make sure that the weight is difficult if the weight is not at least slightly difficult than you're wasting your time. With 15 minutes of kettlebell training plus obeying the sprint diet you can lose a significant amount of weight fast. To learn more about kettlebell training check out my other book "The Kettlebell Cleanse" coming soon.

What's Your Motivation

Now I'm not going to lie to you this type of exercise is incredibly difficult. It's quick and to the point but it's difficult. A lot of people are going to give up because this s*** is probably the hardest form of exercise that your ever going to do. The number one benefit is it's not time consuming. The number two benefit is it's incredibly effective it's the most effective form of exercise on the planet. Nothing will challenge your body more. Nothing will sculpt your body more. Nothing will change your internal chemistry more. This is what makes it the best exercise in the world. Once you start doing it you won't want to stop. It'll become like a drug trust me I'm addicted to this shit. Still getting started will be difficult because your body won't be use to exerting so much energy. The amount of stress that it puts on your energy reserves is amazing but that's what makes you stronger and more energetic. You have to destroy your body so that it can rebuild itself stronger and better. Your body likes to adapt as quickly as it possibly can. This is why exercise eventually becomes easy to you. Your body will adapt to the different complex movements that are involved in aerobic exercise and some forms of weight lifting as well. The only exercise that your body can't get use to is sprinting because it's the one exercise that completely over taxes the body. That means as long as you sprint there will always be progression. All you have to do is add more time but only seconds not hours. Still even knowing this when you actually get up and do it your going to realize what I'm talking about this s*** is no walk in the park. This is for people that are serious about changing their health. Overall aerobic exercise like the treadmill, the elliptical, or the bike will definitely help you in the long run but sprinting changes your health on another level it extends your life without taking away so much of it. Other exercises are literally going to add up to days and months of your life because they're time-consuming there's hours involved. When you look back over your life you're going to realize that a large majority of it was spent just working out when really all you needed was two minutes and 30 seconds. Three minutes and 30 seconds if you're a pro.

You need to find your motivation right now! Did you recently get dumped and you want to create that revenge body that says hey you f***** up? Did you recently get diagnosed with high blood pressure and you want to make sure that you're here to see another day? Did you recently get diagnosed with diabetes and you want to make sure your family doesn't have to bury you before your time? Do you have absolutely no energy whatsoever and it's making your life a living hell? Or do you just want to be sexy as f***? No matter which one of these things applies to you sprinting will help you with it. More energy, better health, better sex, and better looks you can't beat that. Not to mention enhanced strength, speed, and focus. You might as well call this s*** the Superman workout. Just remember whatever your motivation is let that s*** sink down deep within you don't let it go. Let it guide you let it take over you because if you reach the point where it becomes too difficult and you say it's not worth it you'll realize your motivation wasn't strong enough. You need to be motivated you need to be consumed by your reasoning for this otherwise you will give up.

One thing that I love about the Sprint Diet is you can look down on all the other bullshit workouts that your friends are doing. You can look down on all the bullshit you see people in the gym doing because once you start doing this you'll realize that shit is easy. You'll start to see yourself as a real athlete and start looking at those other guys in the gym as lite weights. What they're doing isn't nearly as hard as this. That sense of pride will guide you and push you even further it'll make you feel like you're the s*** and sometimes that's all we need. Sometimes the best motivation on the planet is feeling like you're the s***. My motivation was pretty much every fucking thing on that list. I had high blood pressure. I was pre-diabetic. I had just got dumped and I wanted to be sexy as f***. Those things were ingrained in me. That's all I could think about every single day. I was fixated on it to the point where it became an extreme obsession. The obsessive nature of my thinking was the source of my motivation it pushed me forward every single day. I didn't want high blood pressure because I wanted to make sure that I stayed around to see how the world unfolded. I definitely didn't want diabetes because my grandma died of diabetes and watching her go through that was one of the most excruciating things I've ever dealt with. I had absolutely no energy whatsoever. I could barely stand up without feeling tired. I was always tired. I was always cranky. I was always annoyed with everything. That's how you feel when you have no energy. You feel like everything sucks. You don't want to go anywhere. You don't want to do anything. You don't want to see anyone. You just want to rest. Still no matter how much you rest you still feel tired. It was a horrible experience! Most of all I just wanted to be sexy as f*** I know that sounds a little shallow but at the end of the day we all want to be sexy. We don't want to admit it to anyone else s*** we don't even want to admit it to ourselves. Everyone wants to be sexy, beautiful, attractive whatever the hell you want to call it you want it and you can have it for the low price of 2 minutes and 30 seconds of hard work.

Vitamin Intake

Let me start this off by saying that by no means am I telling you to buy any of these vitamins I'm just telling you the vitamins that I used during the Sprint Diet. I have no idea if they had an effect on my results but I feel like they're worth mentioning. My vitamin intake during the Sprint Diet was well rounded. I tried to make sure I covered every single function of my body. Let's start things off with the first vitamin I took.

Ubiquinol is said to be very good for your cardiovascular health and the last thing I wanted going out on me was my heart because I had high blood pressure. Ubiquinol was a supplement I took to make sure I had a little extra energy. Its supposed to be an incredibly powerful antioxidant it's also supposed to promote energy production as well and I needed all the energy that I could get. They say it's good for brain health and protecting the cells from free radicals. To be honest I still use ubiquinol it's much better than Co q-10 because it's easily absorb into the body.

The second thing I kind of supplemented with was apple cider vinegar with mother. I mixed my apple cider vinegar with a teaspoon of lemon juice, eight ounces of water, and made sure to take this every single day at least 2 times a day. I have no idea what kind of effect it may have had on my progression. I just know that it's still apart of my routine to this day. Apple cider vinegar is supposed to promote weight loss. I have no idea if it contributed to my weight loss but I feel like it's worth mentioning.

The third supplement that I used was black seed oil. Black seed oil is supposed to be the God of all supplements. It's supposed to promote health across the board. They say that it's a huge anti-inflammatory and since pretty much every health problem is caused by inflammation black seed oil is probably the number one vitamin you can use. They say black seed oil is wonderful for cancer prevention and treatment. They also say it's crucial to liver health. They say that it prevents diabetes. They also say it's great for weight loss which was one of the main reasons why I started using it. They say that it's great for your hair, nails, and skin. They also say that it's wonderful for fighting off infections and that it's effective against certain strains of superbugs that most antibiotics are not working on anymore. Black seed oil has been studied over and over again. It's probably one of the most studied supplements on the market so there's some solid science to back up what it does. Still I have no idea if it had a major effect on my workout or not nor do I have any idea if it helped my weight loss.

Another supplement I used was grapeseed, green tea, and pine bark complex. The combination of these created a super antioxidant but the main reason why I was taking it was for energy. The combination of these three things promotes a natural boost in energy. It's not like a caffeine pill or anything like that it's something that works overtime. This is one of those supplements that I don't like running out of I try to make sure that I keep it in stock as much as I possibly can.

I used probiotics because they support your immune system. They're supposed to introduce positive bacteria back into your stomach, which also is supposed to help your digestive system and promote weight loss. I can say that I got sick a lot less often once I start taking the probiotics still I started sprinting around the same time so I can't really say which one was super effective against common ailments.

L-Carnitine was one of the first supplements that I started using. It aids in transforming fat into energy, which is the most important process in weight loss and energy production so I knew that I had to get L-Carnitine immediately. Also it's supposed to aid in muscle building as well. It's actually suppose to be one of the main elements of muscle building. A lot of bodybuilders use L-Carnitine and some even say it helps with your overall brain health. Now I don't know if it did any of these things for me I just know during the Sprint Diet I took it everyday.

Omega-3 fish oil is something that I've been taking since I was a kid. It's supposed to support cardiovascular health and cognitive function. Not to mention your immune system, your bone health, and your joint health as well. It's also said to support a healthy mood. I don't know if it does any of these things I just know that my mom has been giving me omega-3 fish oil since I was a kid. It's supposed to be one of the most important vitamins on the planet for preserving your body and promoting overall health.

Vitamin D3 is a supplement I started taking when I realize that I probably wasn't getting enough of it. Vitamin D comes from sun exposure and since I don't really go outside too often I knew that I probably was vitamin D3 deficient. Vitamin D3 is supposed to support bone destiny, the immune system, and boost absorption of calcium. It's supposed to support neuromuscular function whatever that means. All I know is vitamin D is very important to the body and if you're not getting enough sunlight than most likely you're not getting enough vitamin D3. Still I have no idea if it had any effect on my performance whatsoever.

Biotin is something that I also supplemented with. It's supposed to be good for your hair, nails, and skin. It's also supposed to support some other viable functions in the body. I guess biotin is one of the key ingredients that your hair needs to grow so that's one of the main reasons why I was supplementing with it. I will say when I started to use it I did notice a difference in my hair quality, nail quality, and the appearance of my skin after about maybe three to four months. Still I'm not sure if that was the sprinting or the biotin or a combination of both.

Sea kelp was something else that I used. It's supposed to be a source of iodine. Iodine is important for thyroid function. The thyroid regulates a huge amount of functions in your body including your hormonal balance. Your hormonal balance has a huge effect on your energy levels, your mood, and also your weight. If your thyroid isn't functioning properly than most likely you're going to have weight issues. They say this is why the Japanese are so skinny because their diet is rich in iodine because they eat so much seaweed. Still I have no idea if it had any effect on my weight loss.

Garcinia Cambogia is supposed to stop your body from creating new fat. It was featured on Dr. Oz a while ago and it's supposed to be proven to actually stop your body from creating new fat. Now I'm not sure if it stopped my body from creating new fat all I know is that it was a part of my everyday regimen.

Of course I took a multi vitamin because that just makes common sense. Everybody probably takes a multi-vitamin I've been taking one since I was a kid so that's always pretty much been apart of my regimen.

African Mango was also something that I included in my supplement regimen. It's supposed to help promote weight loss but there isn't much research behind it to say that it does anything of any kind of significance. Still a lot of people swear by it so I added it to my supplement pile.

I also took L-Theanine and if you're a coffee drinker like me L-Theanine is absolutely essential. It gets rid of that jittery affect that coffee gives you and makes it a smooth high. It also has some other benefits that might be worth mentioning. Apparently in 1964 Japan approved L-Theanine for unlimited use in all foods. L-Theanine has been linked to relieving stress. It's the key ingredient in green tea, which has been linked to relieving stress.

I'm not endorsing any of these vitamins in anyway. I'm just informing you of the supplements I used during the Sprint Diet. These supplements may have enhanced my results and it wouldn't be fair if I didn't mention them. If you choose to take them my best advice is to have a conversation with your doctor. If you want to know the exact supplements that I used than check out my website http://workoutkingrule.blogspot.com/.

Mind Your Diet

If you don't pay attention to what the f*** you eat you're not going to be able to accomplish anything. In this situation I'm speaking about eating for energy not eating for weight loss. Remember sprinting takes up a large amount of energy within the body so if you're not eating for a machine than you're not going to be able to sprint for very long. Your body is going to need power so therefore you have to eat the foods that give you the most power. I'm going to give you a detailed example of the type of foods I ate during the Sprint Diet. You can either mimic this or find similar foods that might give you the drive you need.

First thing in the morning I made sure to blend a shake. I blended kale, oranges, apples, bananas, blueberries, cranberries, strawberries, and I used apple juice instead of water. I did research on each one of these fruits and vegetables to make sure that they would give me the optimum performance that I was seeking.

Kale is the healthiest vegetable you can eat because of that I made sure to put more kale in my shake than anything else. Every single fruit that I mention I used a whole one like I used a whole orange, a whole apple, and ah whole banana. I used about maybe eight cranberries, eight blueberries, and about four strawberries. To be honest after I took the shake in the morning I always would feel wonderful. It was probably the best part of my diet and a great way to kick off my day. I also had oatmeal because I wanted to make sure that I was getting an extreme amount of fiber.

The combination of these fruits and vegetables gave me an extreme amount of energy. It's probably the one thing that I can attest to my newfound power. It actually boosts my energy level. I don't know if any of my vitamins did anything to actually boost my energy level but I'm sure my shake did the job especially in combination with oatmeal. To be honest over time it became even more effective. Most people don't understand that eating healthy is something that takes time to affect your body. Sometimes you'll be able to feel it right away but a lot of people quit because they don't feel any difference within a few days or a week. I noticed after a month of taking the shake my overall mood in general changed. Remember I told you I was a very tired, cranky, and moody individual. I was so overweight my body had absolutely no energy whatsoever. When your body has no energy it pretty much ruins everything. You don't want to do anything. I can say that this shake had a profound effect on that mindset and was a key ingredient in making the Sprint Diet much more effective. I made sure that I didn't add any sugar to the mix and I also made sure to put cinnamon in my oatmeal and I found out that actually had a profound effect or my health as well. Remember cinnamon is nothing but pure fiber and fiber is incredibly important to the digestive system. As long as you're going to the bathroom often you're losing weight so you want to make sure you're getting as much fiber as you possibly can. That's why I added apples to the mix because apples are rich in fiber. It's also why I added blueberries to the mix because they're rich in fiber as well. I wanted to make sure that I upped my fiber intake by as much as I possibly could. I also wanted to make sure I was getting a ton of vitamin C.

Vitamin C is the reason why I made sure to add a whole Orange. I added bananas to the mix because I wanted to make sure that I was getting a lot of potassium but really I wanted the bananas for the Vitamin B6. Vitamin B6 is something that you'll see in almost every natural energy supplement.

Cranberries were just another source of fiber they have even more fiber than blueberries they're also packed full of antioxidants. The strawberries were mostly for flavor at first until I started doing more research and I realize that strawberries were amazing. They can help prevent heart disease, stroke, cancer, high blood pressure, constipation, allergies, asthma diabetes, and depression. Strawberries are ah incredibly effective antioxidant.

Oatmeal is packed full of iron it's probably one of the most iron rich foods out there. It also has an extremely large amount of vitamin B6, magnesium, and vitamin A not to mention 6 grams of protein. Speaking of protein maybe I should discuss what I had for lunch.

Everyday for lunch I would have grilled chicken, beans, and a protein shake. My lunch was all about protein intake. At lunch time I wanted to make sure that I was getting as much protein in my body as possible that's why I made sure I had grilled chicken because chicken has an extremely large amount of protein. Chicken is one of the most protein rich meats on the planet and it's healthier for you than beef or pork. Not to mention it's a lot easier to cook especially if you know how to bake or if you have a griller like one of those commercial grillers that drain out all the grease. Everyday when I woke up in the morning I would make sure that I put on my rice cooker and I would add one cup or two cups of black beans. I chose black beans because they're low in calories. One cup is only 624 calories and because they are extremely high in dietary fiber, you get 29 grams in one cup. Also because they're high in protein you get 39 grams of protein in one cup. They have an extremely large amount of iron, and ah extremely large amount of magnesium, and calcium so it was an obvious choice. Black beans are a incredibly healthy super food with 2760 mg of potassium.

The body is supposed to consume at least 30 to 38 grams of fiber every day if you're a man. If you're a woman it's about 25 grams of fiber everyday. So basically one cup of black beans would almost be enough fiber for the day for a man and more than enough for a woman. If you read up on black beans you'll understand just how nutritious they really are. It's one of the most underestimated super foods on the planet. The only substitute that I would ever use for black beans if I didn't have them is quinoa because it's probably the greatest food on the planet and the only food that has pretty much all the amino acids that you need.

I made sure that I had a whey protein isolate shake everyday. Since sprinting increases protein synthesis by 230 percent. Consuming ah s*** ton of protein and sprinting is genius. It's a final trump card to make sure that your body is burning fat and building muscle

For dinner I ate pretty much anything I wanted I just made sure that I didn't eat any fast food. I completely cut out fast food in general. For dinner I would have a meal with black beans on the side. I would have ground turkey meat, chicken, or fish. I wouldn't have any beef or pork. So I would have some turkey tacos with black beans, and cheese, or I would have some turkey nachos with black beans, and cheese. Sometimes I would eat some salmon, beans, and rice. As long as I added the black beans to the meal I would pretty much create any combination I wanted. Eating beans with your meal helps the digestive process not to mention it increases the nutritional value of the meal. I didn't really eat any dessert but I've never been one to eat dessert anyway so it wasn't a big change for me.

My diet wasn't too extreme it wasn't anything that was impractical. All my food was good it wasn't like I had to eat nasty s*** that I didn't like. When you have to eat a bunch of nasty s*** that you don't like eventually you're going to give up on it. I loved the s*** I was eating! My shake was delicious and my oatmeal was always good especially once I added cinnamon. I never put sugar in my oatmeal I just added cinnamon to it. If I wanted it to taste good I would add some honey. I made sure that I got my honey from the whole food store so that my s*** was natural. I didn't mind the beans I was eating because I was eating black beans and those are my favorite especially once you season them with some Lawry's and some pepper. The grilled chicken was always good because I mean grilled chicken is f****** awesome. Sometimes I would grill chicken and have a chicken black bean salad. That s*** was good. My diet gave me energy, power, and change my mood all together. It's the main reason why I was able to go on. If I never changed my diet I would have never saw any positive effects from the Sprint Diet in the first place because I wouldn't be able to do it. My intention was never to change my diet for weight loss but to promote energy production. I simply wanted to feel better and run longer and this diet accomplished that for me. I didn't find it difficult. If you can find food that has similar nutritious value that you actually find delicious by all means go about it in your own way. I'm just telling you exactly what I did I don't want to leave any details out because that might be the one detail that contributed to my progression. If you choose to follow my diet to the letter it is more likely that you will see the same results that I did. Maybe you might find some loopholes that I didn't find and you might be able to improve upon the diet. If so please don't hoard information comment and add your perspective. Tell the people of the dietary changes you implement that worked in combination with the Sprint Diet or maybe some of the vitamins that you used in combination with the Sprint Diet. Share other forms of sprinting that you tried in combination with the Sprint Diet that worked for you.

In Conclusion

    Throughout my workout journey I tried everything in extremes. Some days I would get on the bike for an hour. Than after that I would get on the treadmill for an hour. Than after that I would get on the elliptical for an hour. I did this for months with no results. I decided to get on the elliptical for 3 hours a day making sure that I burned 3000 calories every single day. I did that for a month with no major results. I decided to up the ante and add an extra hour to the equation making sure that I was burning 3500 calories a day and after a month of doing that I saw absolutely no results. 3500 calories is a pound and I wasn't over eating in any way whatsoever. I even boosted it up to five hours on the elliptical everyday and still I got no results. I got so used to doing extended aerobic exercise that I had the energy of a marathon runner. As far as my stamina was concerned my normal day-to-day energy was still low but my ability to keep going on the elliptical machine was impressive yet it got me no major results. I was doing five hours on the elliptical machine burning upwards of 4200 calories and still I saw no results. If I was doing that much work and still not seeing any results imagine ah individual who comes in the gym and does 30 minutes on the bike every single day expecting to see major results. Imagine ah individual who comes in and walks on the treadmill for 45 minutes to an hour and expects to see major results. Imagine someone who comes in and uses the elliptical for an hour and expects to see major results it's unfathomable it's a fantasy. None of those people truly are going to lose any weight. I was out doing everyone in my gym. People were asking me how long I was on the machine because others would tell them that I was there when they arrived and I was there when they left. I was there all day and all night because I was serious about my weight loss. Still it had absolutely no major effects whatsoever the only thing it did was give me the ability to run from one city to the next without getting tired but my body still looked horrible. What's the point of gaining long-term stamina if your body still looks like s***? It was a complete and utter waste of time. If I would have just sprinted from the very beginning I would've had even more stamina long-term, short-term, and day-to-day energy. Not to mention muscle and actually physically visible results, which is what I really, wanted. I wanted physically visible results and that's what sprinting gave me. I could look in the mirror and actually see the inches drop off of me. When I was on the elliptical machine and all the other machines for hours upon hours the only thing I would do is weigh myself on the scale once every 7 days. Admittedly this is a mistake never count on a scale to measure how much you weigh because a scale does not account for how much of your body is muscle and how much of your body is fat and how much of your body is water so it's going to be off it's always going to be off. You measure your weight loss in inches. Get a measuring tape and measure your waistline. The smaller your waist gets the more weight you actually lost and the more muscle you've added to your body. This is a lesson I also had to learn the hard way. Aerobic exercise is good for long-term stamina but it's not efficient at burning fat trust me on this. Like I said before have you ever noticed any of those people that only use the aerobic machines actually lose major weight? Those machines are ancient they've been around since the inception of the gym yet no one speaks of there results being godlike. If those machines were super effective the gym would be much more popular than it is. The most powerful workout tool is sprinting. If more people were sprinting everyday than we would have a much healthier society. Everyone would have much more energy and everyone would waste a lot less time at the gym. I wasted months at the gym trying to push my body as far as I possibly could. I would test the limits of my abilities every single day and yes I was capable of running longer every day but when I looked in the mirror I was looking at the same man. It was frustrating as fuck! To be honest if I wasn't as stubborn as I was I would have stopped doing it a long time ago. The day I discovered sprinting was the day everything changed. From the first run I already knew that this was a type of exercise that really would have a true impact on my weight loss. I knew this type of exercise was going to change the way I felt every day. It's the one type of exercise that I actually respect because I know it's working. I can feel that it is working. I can feel the fatigue. I can feel the endorphins running around in my head. I can feel the rush of dopamine. I can feel my body trying to replenish itself after being taxed to its maximum limit. After every week I could feel the difference in my energy level. This made me feel like I was actually doing something for the first time. I know that sounds crazy because I used to run on an elliptical machine for 5 hours straight but it never taxed my body the way sprinting for 2 minutes did. It was amazing to think that I could move on an elliptical machine with the difficulty turned up almost to max for 5 hours but I could barely sprint 6 times for 10 seconds. This one form of exercise completely changed my life. Everything that I considered motivation for doing this exercise was eventually accomplished. I've never felt better about myself as a person and I've never felt more like I'm the s*** than I do now. Every single day when I get up and look in the mirror I feel like I'm the s***! That doesn't mean that I knock others down or belittle them because I know how it feels to be unconfident and doubtful of your own self-worth. That's why I wrote this book to help people that are doubtful and uncertain of their own self-worth. I wrote this book for people that are on the borderline of giving up because they have tried for so long and have seen absolutely no results whatsoever. It could seem at some point that it's not meant for you to lose weight like your body will never change. That's how I felt before I begun the Sprint Diet. My pre-diabetic status, my high blood pressure, and my low energy all eventually went away by following the principles in this book. If this information can help even one person than it was worth writing down. I've seen tons of information on dieting and exercise throughout the Internet but none of those things helped me. Some people have been skinny their entire lives and than out of nowhere gained a ton of weight and they don't know how to manage it. Weight management is just something that they never had to deal with because their weight was never a concern. Some people have been big their whole life but have never really tried to do anything about it so when they do try they go through this whole list of things that make absolutely no difference. Throughout my journey I listen to many people I took many routes and every one of them led me down the same path. The worst feeling in the world is working as hard as you possibly can at something but literally getting nowhere. It's like the universe is saying your best isn't enough. In the case of exercise it's not that your best isn't enough it's just that you're giving your all to the wrong things. I gave my all to every single form of aerobic exercise you can imagine. Hours every day non-stop spent working out with minimal to no results. Once I gave my all to sprinting I finally could see the fruits of my labor. I finally felt like I actually was doing something productive something beneficial that was pushing past the threshold that I had been at for months. Remember nothing is instantaneous everything takes time but the worst thing you can do is waste your time doing something that isn't beneficial. I'm glad I went down the path I did because now I can invite others to take an alternative route. When I go into the gym and I see people that I know using the treadmill or the elliptical I make sure to inform them that there is an alternative method something more beneficial. I tell them about sprinting and they always think me later. Still I never really felt like I was reaching enough people that way and hopefully through this book I can reach out to people that felt just like I did, willing to make a change but oblivious of how to go about it. We all want to make a change but most of us don't know how to go about it so when we try for the first time and fail some of us never try again. If this is your first time trying to lose weight and become healthy than I'm glad you came here first. Have a good workout and a energetic and long life.